WOMEN WHO THRIVE
GROUP MANUAL
12 UNITS

FAR FROM PERFECT

Women Who Thrive

DON'T GIVE UP
DON'T HOLD IT IN

BY DR. NANCIA LEATH

ISBN 978-0-9796546-6-4

Published in USA by Inward Core, Inc

Table of Content

FAR FROM PERFECT

DON'T GIVE UP

DON'T HOLD IT IN

WWW.WWTHRIVE.COM

WOMEN WHO THRIVE

Group Manual - 12 Units - Dr. Nancia Leath

Introduction

"Friendships are gifts from above to help humans know they are loved and valued." Dr. Nancia Leath

Research shows that having friends in your life is more important than having romantic relationships or having a successful business. It is believed that friends bring more balance in your life than virtually any other relationship. In the Women Who Thrive Community, we want authentic friendships to happen because we understand the huge impact friendships have on your mental health and happiness. Especially when you understand how to develop close friendships and know what you need in a friend. Lacking true friendship connections can lead to depression, anxiety, selfishness, disloyalty, fear of people, lack of relating to others, and lack of emotional maturity. According to Swedish study not having a rich network of friends can also decrease significant years off your life.

Women Who Thrive understand close friendships don't just happen and friendships require sacrifice. Many women struggle with meeting new friends and developing quality connections especially as an adult. Or they may have people they consider their friends, but still feel lonely. Most in this state usually only have once-a-year meet-up with their friends. This cannot be the case if you desire a strong bond. We believe it is important to reconnect with old friends often, but purposely build new relationships to improve your social life, emotional health, and overall well-being. Therefore, Women Who Thrive Connections are very important and needed in order for you to thrive as an individual.

To help you have meaningfully Women Who Thrive Connections, it is important you develop a strong foundation by learning new tools. We believe all Women Who Thrive Connections' foundation need to center around creating healthy relationships. This manual was created to help you with this process. The Women Who Thrive Connections will focus on the importance of developing friendships and tools to maintain relationships among women from different walks of life.

How is this manual to be used?

This manual was created to help guide you through 12 meetings in a small group setting – **limiting participation to 10 to 12 people in each group**. The content of the manual relies on individual members to share their experiences pertaining to their friendships and work through any blockers that will prevent you from thriving. Each unit focuses on different topics and is guided by activities and discussion. This manual was meant to spice up your meetups and help you grow stronger together as you thrive.

What are the goals of this manual?

- For women to receive tools to help develop authentic relationships among women from all walks of life.
- For women to develop tools to empower them to thrive in all areas of their life.
- For women to use as a guide to make sure they are implementing The Women Who Thrive 3 C(s) – Connection, Community, and Collaboration.

Who is this manual for?

This manual was created for all women.

What can I expect from engaging in this process?

You will learn how to accept women for existing and not devalue their worth because of your different perspectives, cultures, race, roles, career, age, etc.

You will be challenged to listen and understand more instead of judging. This will cause your worldview to expand.

What will be required of me?

Commitment to the women in your group and to the process.
Listen with compassion.
Speak to be heard.
Be transparent.
Expect constructive criticism and encouragement.
Be open to explore others' past without judgement.

How can I lead a Women Who Thrive small group or be a Women Who Thrive Connection Leader?

1. **Complete Women Who Thrive Connection Leader legal documentation** – go to our website at www.wwthrive.com and click on "Tell Me More" or copy and paste this link https://forms.gle/eZEbbD4d3EP4w3Pa8.
2. Add a co-leader to assist you and make sure she also completes the Women Who Thrive Connection Leader legal documentation.
3. Plan all events for your group by using this manual.
4. Email info@wwthrive to inform of the location of your group.

FRIENDSHIPS

Welcome to Women Who Thrive Connections

We are so excited you have decided to join Women Who Thrive and your wiliness to build authentic relationships with other women. Expect to meet and network with women from all walks of life to learn from and grow with as you build strong friendships. How? By implementing the Women Who Thrive 3 C(s): Connection, Community, and Collaboration. Get ready for a wonderful ride as you do what it takes to do and be a Woman Who Thrive!

To help you have meaningfully Women Who Thrive Connections, it is important you develop a strong foundation by learning new tools.

WOMEN WHO THRIVE

Group Manual - 12 Units - Dr. Nancia Leath

FRIENDSHIPS

Unit 1: Women Who Thrive - Friendships

Type of Event: Luncheon (You decide location – it can be formal or informal)

Prepare for meeting:
Next meeting time, date, and location for 2nd meeting (look at description for second meeting below to help you decide)
4 door prizes

Agenda for Meeting:

Women Who Thrive Connection Leader:
1. **Welcome Everyone**
2. **Women Who Thrive Purpose:** The purpose for Women Who Thrive is to provide women of all walks of life tools to thrive in all areas of their lives.
3. **Vision Statement:** One day, all women in this nation will have the opportunity to network with other women from all walks of life and thrive. Mission Statement: To inspire healthier communities by connecting women together to collaborate regardless of their differences.
4. **State History:** Women Who Thrive was founded by Dr. Nancia Leath on December 1, 2019. Dr. Leath wanted to give $100 away to help another woman thrive, so she started a group on Facebook and invited friends. She informed everyone that people who invited the most people will receive the $100 in 31 days. Women Who Thrive reached 8000 by December 31, 2019 and it's still growing. There are currently 56 out of 195 countries represented. Women Who Thrive provides by-weekly grants. Women Who Thrive encourage women to meet in small group format to make sure they create authentic relationships and everyone is heard. Women Who Thrive provides trainings within their private Facebook group to help them gain tools to thrive. Since Women Who Thrive is just getting started, you will always be a part of the history because you are another Woman Who Thrives!
5. Ask everyone to post a picture of this event on social media to use #womenwhothrive (5 minutes).

First Connection
Most relationships you build online will not be sustained over the long haul via just social media, for several reasons. It's very easy to misunderstand the intent of what's being said; sometimes it's even difficult to determine context online. It's also very easy not to give 100% in the relationship because you don't have to give your full attention. Even if you don't do it on purpose, it's easy to slip into the habit of reading your emails, chatting with others, or doing online shopping. while also interacting on social media.

Face-to-face interactions are so much different because you're truly more intentional. You turn off your phone or put it on silent, sit back, and listen to the other person. You ask probing questions and wait for them to work out the long, involved, and deeply thought out answers. You can learn from their body language, their facial expressions, and their verbal habits. The relationships you build with people you meet face-to-face are more personal, more real. You spend time getting to know one another, asking about family, hobbies, goals, etc. It's where the true intimacy starts. Today, when you mingle with these women for the first time think about why you want to build a real relationship with them. Why you are willing to commit to the relationship, even after knowing you will have to work through your differences and misunderstandings. Having strong people skills are important to have in order to thrive. You will improve in this area regardless of where you are by purposely meeting together with your Women Who Thrive Connections.

Time: 5 minutes
Number of Participants: Any
Tools Needed: None
Rules: Have each individual walk around and share what they hope to contribute to the Women Who Thrive connections/meetups with as many people as possible. If you want, offer a prize for the person who can tell you at least what 5 people hope to contribute to the Women Who Thrive Connections.
Objective: Improves meeting productivity and makes attendees think about how they're going to contribute, rather than just what they hope to get out of the Women Who Thrive Connections.

Eat meal (15 minutes – give out door prices during this time to keep the energy up**)**
Speaker: The Importance of Friendship – Founder Dr. Nancia Leath or Director of Women Who Thrive Connection Leaders Alexandra Bates (15 minutes)
Meet New People Game (Dr. Leath): This game will allow everyone to spend quality time with at least half the people in attendance. (15 minutes)

Purpose for Women Who Thrive Connection Leader (Dr. Leath):
Purpose for Women Who Thrive Connection Leader
Q&A

Closure (Women Who Thrive Connection Leader)
- Will inform the date, location, and activity for the next meeting.
- Thank everyone for coming.
- Make sure a Group Picture is taken and posted in Women Who Thrive Group on FB
- Encourage group members to buy Women Who Thrive Tee-shirts - www.wwthrive.com.
- Post Pictures within the Women Who Thrive Facebook community tag #womenwhothrive

FRIENDSHIPS

Unit 2: Women Who Thrive – Your Truth

Type of Event: Relationship Building (Connection/Community) – Please have refreshments to serve during the activity (have everyone pay $5 to go towards) or encourage everyone to bring their own/potluck.

Agenda:

Women Who Thrive Connection Leader – Women Who Thrive Connection Leader:

1. **Welcome Everyone**
2. **Women Who Thrive Purpose:** The purpose for Women Who Thrive is to provide women of all walks of life tools to thrive in all areas of their lives.
3. **Vision Statement:** One day, all women in this nation will have the opportunity to network with other women from all walks of life and thrive.
4. **Mission Statement:** To inspire healthier communities by connecting women together to collaborate regardless of their differences.
5. **State History:** Women Who Thrive was founded by Dr. Nancia Leath on December 1, 2019. Dr. Leath wanted to give $100 away to help another woman thrive, so she started a group on Facebook and invited friends. She informed everyone that people who invited the most people will receive the $100 in 31 days. Women Who Thrive reached 8000 by December 31, 2019 and it's still growing. There are currently 56 out of 195 countries represented. Women Who Thrive encourage women to meet in small group format to make sure they create authentic relationships and everyone is heard. Women Who Thrive provides trainings within their private Facebook group to help them gain tools to thrive. Since Women Who Thrive is just getting started, you will always be a part of the history because you are another Woman Who Thrives!
6. Ask everyone to post a picture of this event on social media to use #womenwhothrive (5 minutes).

Truth and Untruths

To help people commit to improve self and respect others it is great for them to learn and talk about self by learning truth and lies. This activity will help people open up. Teams gather together in an intimate environment. Each team member says four truths and two lies about himself. Team members must guess the two lies out of the four statements.

Number of participants: 2-13

Duration: 1 hour

Objective: Break the ice and get people involved

Rules

1. Ask everyone to sit in a circle.

2. Each Women Who Thrive attendant must think of four truths and two lies about herself.

3. Each player then gets up in the center of the circle and says six statements about herself (four truths, two lies).

4. The rest of the group must guess which of the statements is a truth, which one were lies.

5. The process repeats for all other players.

6. Then you will discuss as an entire group all these questions to help build on your relationships.
    1. Why you selected your truths and lies?
    2. Was it easier to create the lies than tell your truth?
    3. Were you able to look the women in their eyes when you told your lies?
    4. Did you judge women based off their lies or truths if so, why? If not why?
    5. What did you learn about each person in the group based off their truth and lies?
    6. What are you willing to do or tell and be your truth when you come together as a group?
    7. What will you need from the ladies in order to put or keep your walls down to maintain solid relationships?

Strategy

There is no competitive element to this activity. Instead, it's designed to get people to open up and get to know each other better. The opportunity to lie can also get some hilariously outrageous statements from players, which further improves the group's mood.

- Closure: The Women Who Thrive Connection Leader will inform the date, location, and activity for the next meeting. Thank everyone for coming.
- Make sure a Group Picture is taken and posted in Women Who Thrive Group
- Encourage group members to buy Women Who Thrive Tee-shirts - www.wwthrive.com.
- Encourage members to post pictures within the Women Who Thrive Facebook community

Unit 3: Women Who Thrive – Life List

Type of Event: Relationship Building (Connection)– Please have refreshments to serve during the activity (have everyone pay $5 to go towards) or encourage everyone to bring their own/potluck.

Agenda:

Women Who Thrive Connection Leader – Women Who Thrive Connection Leader:

1. **Welcome Everyone**
2. **Women Who Thrive Purpose:** The purpose for Women Who Thrive is to provide women of all walks of life tools to thrive in all areas of their lives.
3. **Vision Statement:** One day, all women in this nation will have the opportunity to network with other women from all walks of life and thrive.
4. **Mission Statement:** To inspire healthier communities by connecting women together to collaborate regardless of their differences.
5. **State History:** Women Who Thrive was founded by Dr. Nancia Leath on December 1, 2019. Dr. Leath wanted to give $100 away to help another woman thrive, so she started a group on Facebook and invited friends. She informed everyone that people who invited the most people will receive the $100 in 31 days. Women Who Thrive reached 8000 by December 31, 2019 and it's still growing. There are currently 56 out of 195 countries represented. Women Who Thrive provides by-weekly grants. Women Who Thrive encourage women to meet in small group format to make sure they create authentic relationships and everyone is heard. Women Who Thrive provides trainings within their private Facebook group to help them gain tools to thrive. Since Women Who Thrive is just getting started, you will always be a part of the history because you are another Woman Who Thrives!
6. Ask everyone to post a picture of this event on social media to use #womenwhothrive (5 minutes).

Share Your Life List

If you want to know somebody, you must first know what they want in life. Women Who Thrive will share their Life List, telling each other what matters to them and why. Many are used to creating bucket lists. Bucket lists focus mainly on things you want to do before dying. We are going to focus more on your Life List, which are things you want to do in order to thrive and not just survive. This gives team members a much better understanding of each other's beliefs and motivations than simple personal trivia.

Number of participants: 2+

Duration: 30+ minutes

Objective: Team bonding

Rules:

1. Ask each person to share their top 5 things on her life list. Also, ask everyone to share why it matters to them and how they plan to achieve it. Keep in mind that life lists are meant to be achievable, not outright fantasies ("make a million dollars" is a legitimate goal, "having an elephant in your car" is not).

2. As the participant shares her life list, team members talk about whether any of the items fall on their life list as well, and if yes, why?

3. If two or more participants have the same item on their life lists (happens more than you realize), encourage them to team up and find ways to achieve it together. A shared goal can be a powerful source of team bonding. Decide to do something together as a group on your life list – it could be a mission trip, go on vacation together, or do a cooking video. It honestly doesn't matter what it is, but decide as a group and plan it out!

4. Do this for every participant. You don't have to necessarily follow any structure - just be casual and conversational.

Strategy

Life lists often reveal deep-seated motivations and passions. If you want team members to truly understand each other, sharing their motivations is a great way to help with this process and build real team camaraderie.

- **Closure:** The Women Who Thrive Connection Leader will inform the date, location, and activity for the next meeting. Thank everyone for coming.
- Make sure a Group Picture is taken and posted in Women Who Thrive Group
- Encourage group members to buy Women Who Thrive Tee-shirts - www.wwthrive.com.
- Encourage members to post pictures within the Women Who Thrive Facebook community

Unit 4: Women Who Thrive - Commitment

Type of Event: Commitment (Community)– Please have refreshments to serve during the activity (have everyone pay $5 to go towards) or encourage everyone to bring their own/potluck.

Agenda:

Women Who Thrive Connection Leader – Women Who Thrive Connection Leader:

1. **Welcome Everyone**
2. **Women Who Thrive Purpose:** The purpose for Women Who Thrive is to provide women of all walks of life tools to thrive in all areas of their lives.
3. **Vision Statement:** One day, all women in this nation will have the opportunity to network with other women from all walks of life and thrive.
4. **Mission Statement:** To inspire healthier communities by connecting women together to collaborate regardless of their differences.
5. **State History:** Women Who Thrive was founded by Dr. Nancia Leath on December 1, 2019. Dr. Leath wanted to give $100 away to help another woman thrive, so she started a group on Facebook and invited friends. She informed everyone that people who invited the most people will receive the $100 in 31 days. Women Who Thrive reached 8000 by December 31, 2019 and it's still growing. There are currently 56 out of 195 countries represented. Women Who Thrive provides by-weekly grants. Women Who Thrive encourage women to meet in small group format to make sure they create authentic relationships and everyone is heard. Women Who Thrive provides trainings within their private Facebook group to help them gain tools to thrive. Since Women Who Thrive is just getting started, you will always be a part of the history because you are another Woman Who Thrives!
6. Ask everyone to post a picture of this event on social media to use #womenwhothrive (5 minutes).

Commitment

People often desire interpersonal connections to help them feel wanted, whole, and content. Different people go about this in different ways. You could be a part of Women Who Thrive. To satisfy this craving, you may have to gain true friendships. Please understand that although you may desire interpersonal connections, you may be the reasons why you lack close connections. Research shows that many women have commitment issues, especially with other women. They are quicker to trust a man faster than women in most situations concerning friendships. However, in the workplace, data shows that many prefer to trust women than men. There are many reasons why, but today we are going to focus on your commitment level with maintaining friendships with other women.

Number of participants: 2+

Duration: 30+ minutes

Objective: Commitment bonding

Rules:

1. Ask each person to share the top 2 commitment issues that maybe hurdles that can keep her from forging quality, long-term relationships with other women. Also, ask them to share why it matters to have quality relationships and how do they go about maintaining them. If they don't know how or don't have quality relationships, encourage them to commit to the women in Women Who Thrive Group.

2. As the participant shares her commitment issues, encourage team members to talk about their similarities and how are they willing to work together to overcome their fear of commitment to friendship. If they don't have any fears discuss what they are willing to do to deepen their relationships with others in Women Who Thrive Group. A shared goal can be a powerful source of commitment bonding.

4. Do this for every participant. You don't have to necessarily follow any structure - just be casual and conversational.

Strategy

Telling your commitment issues often reveal deep-seated motivations and conflicts. If you want team members to truly understand each other, sharing these motivations is a great way to break down walls and build real quality relationships.

Closure:
- The Women Who Thrive Connection Leader will inform the date, location, and activity for the next meeting. Thank everyone for coming.
- Make sure a Group Picture is taken and posted in Women Who Thrive Facebook Group.
- Encourage group members to buy Women Who Thrive Tee-shirts - www.wwthrive.com.
- Encourage members to post pictures within the Women Who Thrive Facebook community.

FRIENDSHIPS

Unit 5: Women Who Thrive – Leadership Development

Type of Event: Leadership Development (Collaboration) – Please have refreshments to serve during the activity (have everyone pay $5 to go towards) or encourage everyone to bring their own/potluck.

Agenda:

Women Who Thrive Connection Leader – Women Who Thrive Connection Leader:

1. **Welcome Everyone**
2. **Women Who Thrive Purpose:** The purpose for Women Who Thrive is to provide women of all walks of life tools to thrive in all areas of their lives.
3. **Vision Statement:** One day, all women in this nation will have the opportunity to network with other women from all walks of life and thrive.
4. **Mission Statement:** To inspire healthier communities by connecting women together to collaborate regardless of their differences.
5. **State History:** Women Who Thrive was founded by Dr. Nancia Leath on December 1, 2019. Dr. Leath wanted to give $100 away to help another woman thrive, so she started a group on Facebook and invited friends. She informed everyone that people who invited the most people will receive the $100 in 31 days. Women Who Thrive reached 8000 by December 31, 2019 and it's still growing. There are currently 56 out of 195 countries represented. Women Who Thrive provides by-weekly grants. Women Who Thrive encourage women to meet in small group format to make sure they create authentic relationships and everyone is heard. Women Who Thrive provides trainings within their private Facebook group to help them gain tools to thrive. Since Women Who Thrive is just getting started, you will always be a part of the history because you are another Woman Who Thrives!
6. Ask everyone to post a picture of this event on social media to use #womenwhothrive (5 minutes)

Leadership Development

This activity will show you what it means to collaborate. You will rely heavily on problem solving and leadership skills. Some team members might stand out and some might stand back, but it's important to remember that the entire team must come to a consensus before a decision is made.

Number of participants: 5+

Duration: 1 -2 hours

Objective: Leadership Development

Tools Needed: Different jigsaw puzzles for each group

Rules:

1. Have everyone break off into small, equal-sized groups. Give each group a different jigsaw puzzle with the same difficulty level. The goal is to see which group can complete their jigsaw puzzle the fastest. However, some pieces will be mixed around in other group's jigsaw puzzles. It's up to the team to come up with a way to get those pieces back — either through negotiating, trading, exchanging team members, etc. Whatever they decide to do, they must decide as a group.
2. Discuss together at the end of what approaches were used to get the pieces back. What worked and what did not work? How can you use what you learned in your relationships to help build your life puzzle or in your homes in order to maintain unity and completing projects or reaching goals?

Strategy

This activity will rely heavily on problem solving and leadership skills. Some team members might stand out and some might stand back, but it's important to remember that the entire team must come to a consensus before a decision is made.

Closure
- The Women Who Thrive Connection Leader will inform the date, location, and activity for the next meeting. Thank everyone for coming.
- Make sure a Group Picture is taken and posted in Women Who Thrive Facebook Group.
- Encourage group members to buy Women Who Thrive Tee-shirts - www.wwthrive.com.
- Encourage members to post pictures within the Women Who Thrive Facebook community.

Unit 6: Women Who Thrive —Identity

Type of Event: Self-Development (Connection/Community) – Please have refreshments to serve during the activity (have everyone pay $5 to go towards) or encourage everyone to bring their own/potluck.

Agenda:

Women Who Thrive Connection Leader – Women Who Thrive Connection Leader:

1. **Welcome Everyone**
2. **Women Who Thrive Purpose:** The purpose for Women Who Thrive is to provide women of all walks of life tools to thrive in all areas of their lives.
3. **Vision Statement:** One day, all women in this nation will have the opportunity to network with other women from all walks of life and thrive.
4. **Mission Statement:** To inspire healthier communities by connecting women together to collaborate regardless of their differences.
5. **State History:** Women Who Thrive was founded by Dr. Nancia Leath on December 1, 2019. Dr. Leath wanted to give $100 away to help another woman thrive, so she started a group on Facebook and invited friends. She informed everyone that people who invited the most people will receive the $100 in 31 days. Women Who Thrive reached 8000 by December 31, 2019 and it's still growing. There are 56 out of 195 countries represented. Women Who Thrive provides by-weekly grants. Women Who Thrive encourage women to meet in small group format to make sure they create authentic relationships and everyone is heard. Women Who Thrive provides trainings within their private Facebook group to help them gain tools to thrive. Since Women Who Thrive is just getting started, you will always be a part of the history because you are another Woman Who Thrives!
6. Ask everyone to post a picture of this event on social media to use #womenwhothrive (5 minutes)

Explain Your Identity

This activity will help you explain your identity to others and express what you do to help you enter new circles to help you grow as an individual. An identity is not a fixed thing. It is constantly changing and being molded by your experiences. If you have recently gone through something that has made you question how you are living your life, it can leave you feeling at odds with the person you currently see when you look in the mirror.

Number of participants: 2+

Duration: 1 hours

Objective: Self-Development

Tools Needed: Purchase several index cards, enough for each participant to have ten index cards (for example, if you have sixteen players, you need at least 160 cards). Also purchase pens so that each participant has one to use.

Rules:

1. Hand out the index cards and pens to each participant. Ask the participants to think about their values and what makes up their identity. Instruct them to write one value on each index card. They should have written down 10 values in total.
2. Once everyone has their values written down, have the participants share with their first partner why they chose to write down those values. After sharing for 5-7 minutes, ask all participants to rip up one of their cards that they less prioritize. This part of the activity gives participants an opportunity to reflect on how they prioritize their values. Ripping up the card should help the participant imagine living without that part of their identity. After the participants rip up one card, the outer circle will rotate one partner to the right. Everyone should have a new partner now. Have the new pairs discuss why they ripped up the card they ripped up.
3. Continue this process until all participants are each left with one card — their most important value. Have everyone discuss why this particular value is important and why they can't live without this value.
4. As a group discuss the times you have been judged for thinking and looking differently and moments you have judged others for not agreeing with what you valued.
5. Discuss why is it important to seek to understand others more than trying to get people to agree with your view points.
6. What will you like to change about yourself or your values after hearing others' values?
7. Now place all your cards that are left so all can view and ask these questions: What do these values say about us as a group? Are there similarities? Are there some that surprise you? Are there values you have questions about?

Strategy

This activity will help you identify what values are important to you and what values you will like to add in your life. You will also learn about what others consider important concerning their values.

Closure:
- The Women Who Thrive Connection Leader will inform the date, location, and activity for the next meeting. Thank everyone for coming.
- Make sure a Group Picture is taken and posted in Women Who Thrive Facebook Group.
- Encourage group members to buy Women Who Thrive Tee-shirts - www.wwthrive.com.
- Encourage members to post pictures within the Women Who Thrive Facebook community.

FRIENDSHIPS

Unit 7: Women Who Thrive – Old Story

Type of Event: Self-Development (Community/Connection) – Please have refreshments to serve during the activity (have everyone pay $5 to go towards) or encourage everyone to bring their own/potluck.

Agenda:

Women Who Thrive Connection Leader – Women Who Thrive Connection Leader:

1. **Welcome Everyone**
2. **Women Who Thrive Purpose:** The purpose for Women Who Thrive is to provide women of all walks of life tools to thrive in all areas of their lives.
3. **Vision Statement:** One day, all women in this nation will have the opportunity to network with other women from all walks of life and thrive.
4. **Mission Statement:** To inspire healthier communities by connecting women together to collaborate regardless of their differences.
5. **State History:** Women Who Thrive was founded by Dr. Nancia Leath on December 1, 2019. Dr. Leath wanted to give $100 away to help another woman thrive, so she started a group on Facebook and invited friends. She informed everyone that people who invited the most people will receive the $100 in 31 days. Women Who Thrive reached 8000 by December 31, 2019 and it's still growing. There are 56 out of 195 countries represented. Women Who Thrive provides by-weekly grants. Women Who Thrive encourage women to meet in small group format to make sure they create authentic relationships and everyone is heard. Women Who Thrive provides trainings within their private Facebook group to help them gain tools to thrive. Since Women Who Thrive is just getting started, you will always be a part of the history because you are another Woman Who Thrives!
6. Ask everyone to post a picture of this event on social media to use #womenwhothrive (5 minutes)

Your Old Story

This activity will allow you to change your old story to your future story. Many of you take time to focus on what will go wrong and not what will go right in friendships. Your past is no longer your current story, but your old story. Today, identify what you want your future story to be. Your future is the next second, hour, day, month, or year.

Number of participants: 2+

Duration: 1 hours

Objective: Self-Development

Tools Needed: Paper, pen, and color pencils.

Rules:

1. Hand out the paper and pens to each participant. Ask the participants to think about what they want their future to be concerning their friendships.
2. Once everyone has their future for friendship written down, divide everyone into groups of two. Have the two individuals sitting back-to-back
3. Give one person the pen and paper and the other person describes their future friendships. The person with their story describes to their teammate for her to draw the future of the person. The person with the pen and paper draws what they think the person is saying, based on the verbal description. Then switch roles. Set a time limit for 10 - 15 minutes.
4. Switch roles to make sure everyone have a chance to draw and describe their future friendships.
5. Question to ask the group: Now that you have spoken about values in our last meeting, what will you need to do to help you take steps to become your future indicated in this activity?

Strategy

This is an activity that focuses on interpretation and communication. Once the drawing is finished, it's always interesting to see how the drawer interprets their partner's description. It also allows the person to identify what she wants in a friendship and how others will view it.

Closure:
- The Women Who Thrive Connection Leader will inform the date, location, and activity for the next meeting. Thank everyone for coming.
- Make sure a Group Picture is taken and posted in Women Who Thrive Facebook Group.
- Encourage group members to buy Women Who Thrive Tee-shirts - www.wwthrive.com.
- Encourage members to post pictures within the Women Who Thrive Facebook community.

FRIENDSHIPS

Unit 8: Women Who Thrive – Lift Up

Type of Event: Relationship-Development (Connection/Community) – Please have refreshments to serve during the activity (have everyone pay $5 to go towards) or encourage everyone to bring their own/potluck.

Agenda:

Women Who Thrive Connection Leader – Women Who Thrive Connection Leader:

1. **Welcome Everyone**
2. **Women Who Thrive Purpose:** The purpose for Women Who Thrive is to provide women of all walks of life tools to thrive in all areas of their lives.
3. **Vision Statement:** One day, all women in this nation will have the opportunity to network with other women from all walks of life and thrive.
4. **Mission Statement:** To inspire healthier communities by connecting women together to collaborate regardless of their differences.
5. **State History:** Women Who Thrive was founded by Dr. Nancia Leath on December 1, 2019. Dr. Leath wanted to give $100 away to help another woman thrive, so she started a group on Facebook and invited friends. She informed everyone that people who invited the most people will receive the $100 in 31 days. Women Who Thrive reached 8000 by December 31, 2019 and it's still growing. There are 56 out of 195 countries represented. Women Who Thrive provides by-weekly grants. Women Who Thrive encourage women to meet in small group format to make sure they create authentic relationships and everyone is heard. Women Who Thrive provides trainings within their private Facebook group to help them gain tools to thrive. Since Women Who Thrive is just getting started, you will always be a part of the history because you are another Woman Who Thrives!
6. Ask everyone to post a picture of this event on social media to use #womenwhothrive (5 minutes)

Lift Up

This activity will allow you to understand the consequences of competition and benefits of collaboration. Competition can hold you back from achieving your greatest potential because it is inherently divisive. There can only be one winner. Collaboration, on the other hand, is all about progressing as a whole. There is no winner unless the entire group crosses the finish line together. In Women Who Thrive, we want you to collaborate more instead of competing between each other.

Number of participants: 2+

Duration: 1 hours

Objective: Relationship-Development

Tools Needed: NA

Rules:

1. Discuss why it's important to lift others up instead of competing against others.
2. Discuss moments you had to back down or put someone before you in order to win as a team. Will you be willing to put others before you at different moments if it was needed for the team to grow or become stronger?
3. Discuss when you find yourself wanting to compete with other women and your why.
4. What do you do to collaborate with others in your life now?
5. How will you like to improve in how you collaborate with Women Who Thrive?
6. Discuss how you would like to be encouraged from the Women Who Thrive (please don't ask for money unless it's a serious need). Find out how all of you can help each other thrive in different areas in your life.
7. Decide today to support everyone in your group by posting about their businesses on your social media, sending them referrals, send them encouraging texts, post encouraging content in the Women Who Thrive Group at least 3x a week to help all Women Who Thrive, and/or purposely like what they post.

Strategy

This is an activity that focuses on collaborating more than competing with one another. Plus, implement steps to purposely lift each other up to build genuine relationships.

Closure:
- The Women Who Thrive Connection Leader will inform the date, location, and activity for the next meeting. Thank everyone for coming.
- Make sure a Group Picture is taken and posted in Women Who Thrive Facebook Group.
- Encourage group members to buy Women Who Thrive Tee-shirts - www.wwthrive.com.
- Encourage members to post pictures within the Women Who Thrive Facebook community.

FRIENDSHIPS

Unit 9: Women Who Thrive – Seek to Understand

Type of Event: Relationship-Development (Community/Connection) – Please have refreshments to serve during the activity (have everyone pay $5 to go towards) or encourage everyone to bring their own/potluck.

Agenda:
Women Who Thrive Connection Leader – Women Who Thrive Connection Leader:
1. **Welcome Everyone**
2. **Women Who Thrive Purpose:** The purpose for Women Who Thrive is to provide women of all walks of life tools to thrive in all areas of their lives.
3. **Vision Statement:** One day, all women in this nation will have the opportunity to network with other women from all walks of life and thrive.
4. **Mission Statement:** To inspire healthier communities by connecting women together to collaborate regardless of their differences.
5. **State History:** Women Who Thrive was founded by Dr. Nancia Leath on December 1, 2019. Dr. Leath wanted to give $100 away to help another woman thrive, so she started a group on Facebook and invited friends. She informed everyone that people who invited the most people will receive the $100 in 31 days. Women Who Thrive reached 8000 by December 31, 2019 and it's still growing. There are 56 out of 195 countries represented. Women Who Thrive provides by-weekly grants. Women Who Thrive encourage women to meet in small group format to make sure they create authentic relationships and everyone is heard. Women Who Thrive provides trainings within their private Facebook group to help them gain tools to thrive. Since Women Who Thrive is just getting started, you will always be a part of the history because you are another Woman Who Thrives!
6. Ask everyone to post a picture of this event on social media to use #womenwhothrive (5 minutes)

Seek to Understand

This activity will allow you to seek to understand more than trying to put people in your boxes (your perceptions). Most people rather be understood and do what's needed to get their point across. This usually leads to a disconnection and may cause both parties to feel they are not being heard. Instead of listening to what the other person is saying you are thinking more of how she is incorrect and ignoring completely what she is saying. You act as though you are listening but honestly waiting to prove your point. Today learn a tool and practice implementing how to listen to understand instead of focusing more on being understood.

Number of participants: 2+

Duration: 1 hours

Objective: Relationship-Development

Tools Needed: NA

Rules:

1. Divide the group into two teams.
2. You are going to debate on different topics, but instead of team giving opposing viewpoints they will need to paraphrase what the other team stated and provide 3 to 5 reasons why the other team statements are true instead of disagreeing. **For example:** One Team may say: Relationships are important - The Opposing will say: Relationships are important because are needed to help you thrive as a person. Relationships are important because it shows you all people are different. Relationships are important because we think people should not live their lives alone.
3. Topics: 1) Friendships are needed. 2) Forgiving others is one key components in having a long-lasting relationship. 3) Learning to agree to disagree with respect is a sign of maturity. 4) Apologizing is a sign you value the relationship. 5) It's better to tell the truth even if it leads to conflict. 6) There are many ways to show you support others, but it's best to give support in how they need it and not what you think they need. 7) You are good enough despite your short comings. 8) You are one of a kind.

Strategy

This is an activity that focuses on building rapport with others by purposely seeking to understand, instead of debate or correcting them. Relationships improve when others think they are being heard, you care what they are saying, and they are being understood. This causes them to give you the benefit of the doubt.

Closure
- The Women Who Thrive Connection Leader will inform the date, location, and activity for the next meeting. Thank everyone for coming.
- Make sure a Group Picture is taken and posted in Women Who Thrive Facebook Group.
- Encourage group members to buy Women Who Thrive Tee-shirts - www.wwthrive.com.
- Encourage members to post pictures within the Women Who Thrive Facebook community.

Unit 10: Women Who Thrive – Accept the Differences

Type of Event: Relationship-Development and Communication Skills (Collaboration/Community/Connection) – Please have refreshments to serve during the activity (have everyone pay $5 to go towards) or encourage everyone to bring their own/potluck.

Agenda:

Women Who Thrive Connection Leader – Women Who Thrive Connection Leader:

1. **Welcome Everyone**
2. **Women Who Thrive Purpose:** The purpose for Women Who Thrive is to provide women of all walks of life tools to thrive in all areas of their lives.
3. **Vision Statement:** One day, all women in this nation will have the opportunity to network with other women from all walks of life and thrive.
4. **Mission Statement:** To inspire healthier communities by connecting women together to collaborate regardless of their differences.
5. **State History:** Women Who Thrive was founded by Dr. Nancia Leath on December 1, 2019. Dr. Leath wanted to give $100 away to help another woman thrive, so she started a group on Facebook and invited friends. She informed everyone that people who invited the most people will receive the $100 in 31 days. Women Who Thrive reached 8000 by December 31, 2019 and it's still growing. There are 56 out of 195 countries represented. Women Who Thrive provides by-weekly grants. Women Who Thrive encourage women to meet in small group format to make sure they create authentic relationships and everyone is heard. Women Who Thrive provides trainings within their private Facebook group to help them gain tools to thrive. Since Women Who Thrive is just getting started, you will always be a part of the history because you are another Woman Who Thrives!
6. Ask everyone to post a picture of this event on social media to use #womenwhothrive (5 minutes)

Accept the Differences

This activity will allow you to seek to understand the importance of accepting each other's differences. Accepting someone completely means to learn how to separate their actions/behaviors from how you value them as a person. Most people think they will need to accept negative behaviors to accept someone unconditionally. However, this is not the case because you will be rejecting yourself. To accept someone unconditionally, you decide to value them as a person and refuse to see them as worthless. Yet, you have boundaries in place to protect yourself if that person has actions that will cause you harm physically, mentally, spiritually, or even emotionally. You don't try to change the person, but you do what's needed to protect yourself. You make a sound decision not to be judgmental about their value because of their actions. When you make a sound decision to maintain value for all people, you can agree to disagree with respect.

Number of participants: 2+

Duration: 1 hours

Objective: Relationship-Development and Communication Skills

Tools Needed: Baskets or something to hold objects (it can be a brown paper bag). Each person will need 1 partner, which will be consider 1 team. If you have 10 people you will need only 5 baskets. You will need 12 objects for each team. For an example if you have 10 people you will have 5 teams and you need 60 objects. Set up a play area with several objects like books, water bottles, shoes, etc. around it. The objects must be unique enough that people can differentiate between them by touch alone. Also, place a large basket/bag in the center of the play area.

Communication skills and trust are vital to succeed in this activity. You cannot devalue the person or judge anyone during the process. You will need to listen and value the people who are providing instructions and value the individuals who are receiving your instructions.

Rules:

1. Divide Women Who Thrive Members into teams 2 people teams.
2. One person on each team is blindfolded.
3. The blindfolded person will hear instructions from team member. Then the team member will switch to a different team after giving directions to the blindfolded person to retrieve objects from the playing area.
4. A person not a part of a team will whisper out a random object from the play area for the non-blindfolded group to provide directions to those who are blindfolded (It is important that the blindfolded don't hear the object being told to non-blindfolded group).
5. The blindfolded volunteers from each team must race against a clock (2-3 minutes) to pick up their respective objects and drop them into the basket in the center of the room. They cannot see or ask questions; they must rely entirely on instructions from person providing the directions.
6. The person that's providing the directions cannot name the object; they must first describe the object, its shape and its intended purpose. Then they must instruct the volunteer on how to reach the object and get it to the basket.
7. Repeat the process and make sure the person that's blindfolded hear directions from different people until all the objects are placed into the bag or basket.
8. Remove the blindfold and come together as 1 group.
9. Discuss how the instructions were different from each person and why it was important not to judge the instructions by being the person blindfolded.
10. Discuss how you needed to value the person who were providing the instructions and why it was important you value the person who were blindfolded.
11. Discuss how frustrated it was when the person who was blindfolded did not understand your instructions or picked up the wrong item. Did you want to give up on helping the

person? Did you want to judge the person for not being able to understand your instructions or not getting it in bag/basket fast enough?

Strategy

The blindfold is one of the simplest, yet most effective tools in helping all understand the importance in valuing both parties, regardless of the role played if they wanted to thrive over all. It immediately increases the importance of communication and forces all parties to work together.

Closure:
- The Women Who Thrive Connection Leader will inform the date, location, and activity for the next meeting. Thank everyone for coming.
- Make sure a Group Picture is taken and posted in Women Who Thrive Facebook Group.
- Encourage group members to buy Women Who Thrive Tee-shirts - www.wwthrive.com.
- Encourage members to post pictures within the Women Who Thrive Facebook community.

WOMEN WHO THRIVE

Group Manual - 12 Units - Dr. Nancia Leath

FRIENDSHIPS

Unit 11: Women Who Thrive – Forgiveness Party

Type of Event: Self-Development (Collaboration/Community/Connection) – Please have refreshments to serve during the activity (have everyone pay $5 to go towards) or encourage everyone to bring their own/potluck.

Agenda:

Women Who Thrive Connection Leader – Women Who Thrive Connection Leader:
1. **Welcome Everyone**
2. **Women Who Thrive Purpose:** The purpose for Women Who Thrive is to provide women of all walks of life tools to thrive in all areas of their lives.
3. **Vision Statement:** One day, all women in this nation will have the opportunity to network with other women from all walks of life and thrive.
4. **Mission Statement:** To inspire healthier communities by connecting women together to collaborate regardless of their differences.
5. **State History:** Women Who Thrive was founded by Dr. Nancia Leath on December 1, 2019. Dr. Leath wanted to give $100 away to help another woman thrive, so she started a group on Facebook and invited friends. She informed everyone that people who invited the most people will receive the $100 in 31 days. Women Who Thrive reached 8000 by December 31, 2019 and it's still growing. There are 56 out of 195 countries represented. Women Who Thrive provides by-weekly grants. Women Who Thrive encourage women to meet in small group format to make sure they create authentic relationships and everyone is heard. Women Who Thrive provides trainings within their private Facebook group to help them gain tools to thrive. Since Women Who Thrive is just getting started, you will always be a part of the history because you are another Woman Who Thrives!
6. Ask everyone to post a picture of this event on social media to use #womenwhothrive (5 minutes)

Forgiveness Party

This activity will allow you to seek to understand the importance of expressing how you are feeling and saying you are sorry even if you don't understand why the person felt offended.

Number of participants: 2+

Duration: 1 hours

Objective: Relationship-Development and Communication Skills

Tools Needed: Sticky notes and pen – fire pit (or anything you can use that's safe to burn paper), Burning your post is an illustration of what you should do when forgiving someone. No unfolding it and picking it back up again, but destroying (burning) the offense. Music for dancing and décor for party.

Rules:

1. Give each person a pen and five sticky notes
2. The Women Who Thrive Connection Leader will ask everyone to write down something they may have been offended by or rubbed them the wrong way by someone in the group or outside of the group.
3. On the back of the same sticky note write down why you decided to forgive that person.
4. If someone in the room offended you, take them to the side (not in front of everyone) and let them know you have decided to forgive her and your why.
5. If you are asked to be spoken to by one or more of the ladies, please decide to forgive in-advance and don't become offended. Thank the person for forgiving you before even being aware of the offense.
6. Most women will be tempted to become offended because of shame or pride of being pulled to the side. What you are feeling is normal, but focus more on the purpose and why this is needed instead of the shame or pride. Decide not to talk or gossip about it with others in the group or outside the group. Let it stay right there. State how it made you feel to everyone and why you have decided to also forgive. If you don't want to say it to the group -write a note of how you feel and on the back why you decided to forgive.
7. You will take the sticky notes and burn them in fire pit. This is your sign or demonstration of letting your offenses go.
8. Then play music, eat, and dance – this is your way of celebrating for being free of any offenses and being able to forgive. Your first Forgiveness Party!

Strategy

Forgiving others before they ask you for forgiveness gives you back the power that was taken away when you were offended or caused harm regardless of what happened. This strategy teaches you how to celebrate for having freedom from offenses and harm caused.

Closure:
- The Women Who Thrive Connection Leader will inform the date, location, and activity for the next meeting. Thank everyone for coming.
- Make sure a Group Picture is taken and posted in Women Who Thrive Facebook Group.
- Encourage group members to buy Women Who Thrive Tee-shirts - www.wwthrive.com.
- Encourage members to post pictures within the Women Who Thrive Facebook community.

FRIENDSHIPS

Unit 12: Women Who Thrive – I Belong

Type of Event: Self-Development (Community/Connection/Collaboration) – Please have refreshments to serve during the activity (have everyone pay $5 to go towards) or encourage everyone to bring their own/potluck.

Agenda:

Women Who Thrive Connection Leader – Women Who Thrive Connection Leader:

1. **Welcome Everyone**
2. **Women Who Thrive Purpose:** The purpose for Women Who Thrive is to provide women of all walks of life tools to thrive in all areas of their lives.
3. **Vision Statement:** One day, all women in this nation will have the opportunity to network with other women from all walks of life and thrive.
4. **Mission Statement:** To inspire healthier communities by connecting women together to collaborate regardless of their differences.
5. **State History:** Women Who Thrive was founded by Dr. Nancia Leath on December 1, 2019. Dr. Leath wanted to give $100 away to help another woman thrive, so she started a group on Facebook and invited friends. She informed everyone that people who invited the most people will receive the $100 in 31 days. Women Who Thrive reached 8000 by December 31, 2019 and it's still growing. There are 56 out of 195 countries represented. Women Who Thrive provides by-weekly grants. Women Who Thrive encourage women to meet in small group format to make sure they create authentic relationships and everyone is heard. Women Who Thrive provides trainings within their private Facebook group to help them gain tools to thrive. Since Women Who Thrive is just getting started, you will always be a part of the history because you are another Woman Who Thrives!
6. Ask everyone to post a picture of this event on social media to use #womenwhothrive (5 minutes)

I Belong

This activity will allow you to review your life and think about businesses, places, or people you will like to meet in the future. You will discuss what you can do to help you believe you belong in those roles, locations, or the presences of the people.

Number of participants: 2+

Duration: 1 hours

Objective: Self-Development

Tools Needed: Paper and pen–

Rules:

1. Write down the areas in your life you will like to change.
2. Under each area indicate what was preventing you today from being and having your true desires.
3. Write down why you belong in the areas you desire.
4. Partner with someone you usually don't talk much to in the group of why you belong.
5. Discuss what caused you to believe you didn't belong with a group of people (rich, who hold an office in the community, etc.).
6. Discuss if someone you admired (parents, best friends, or family) ever told you did not belong and how did you counteract their words.
7. Discuss what steps you are going to take to be where you believe you belong. Please understand you must start with your belief system.
8. Let's start now - Write on your paper "I belong_____."
9. All in Women Who Thrive Group say together aloud "Today I will go and be and no longer believe I don't belong_____. Even if I'm afraid or expect rejection, I will (be/go/do) _____. I'm strong and willing to face stumbling blocks. I will not give up. I know I'm far from perfect, which is great, because it helps me keep my trust in God. I give Him permission to lead and guide me. I will think on things that are good and accept who I AM in God. I will always believe I am a Woman Who Thrives!
10. Take the challenge to say quote above for 7 days -2 times a day. This will help you with bending your mind and prevent you from dwelling on fear and negative thinking when they occur.

Strategy

Knowing you belong will help remove fears and help you maintain determination, especially when things get tough in your life and you want to give up. It really doesn't matter what it is, even sickness. You tell yourself you belong and trust God to open a door for you and guide you to a better outcome. Learn how to live in harmony and peace by learning how to control your thoughts and purposely thinking on things that are good. It is important for you to know you belong and who you are as a woman in order to **THRIVE!**

Closure
- The Women Who Thrive Connection Leader will inform the date, location, and activity for the next meeting. Thank everyone for coming.
- Make sure a Group Picture is taken and posted in Women Who Thrive Facebook Group.
- Encourage group members to buy Women Who Thrive Tee-shirts - www.wwthrive.com.
- Encourage members to post pictures within the Women Who Thrive Facebook community.

FRIENDSHIPS

What's Next:

Continue to commit to the principles of this manual by having social gatherings. If you decide as a group to redo this manual please note you may have different responses because of your growth as an individual and increase of trust with others in your group. Women Who Thrive will continue to support your growth as you go into your 2nd year.

Consider informing women at your workplace, churches, sororities, or any organizations you are apart about this manual if they want to become stronger as a group.

Continue to implement grow challenges as a group to help you thrive.

Examples of challenges:
- Attending Women Who Thrive Self-publish training to self-publish your own book.
- Attending one of the Women Who Thrive Leadership Trips/retreat/conference together.
- Walking 100 miles within 100 days as a group.
- Praying for each other's goals/family for 5 days over a conference call.
- Collecting money as a group to donate to Women Who Thrive Grant.
- Completing the seven-day mental or physical diet/fast.

Thank you for investing in yourself and others by completing this manual.

Special Thanks to Kathy Simon, Tange Amouzougan, and Alexandra Bates for volunteering their time to edit this amazing manual.

Deep and meaningful relationships play a vital role in overall well-being.

WOMEN WHO THRIVE

Group Manual - 12 Units - Dr. Nancia Leath

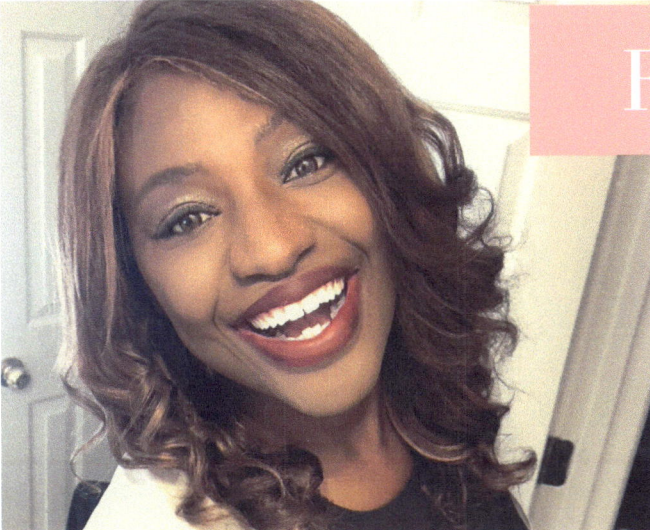

FRIENDSHIPS

This manual was created for women to use as a tool to help develop stronger relationships when they come together in small group settings.

ALL WOMEN

Women Who Thrive Group Manual was created for all women, regardless of their differences.

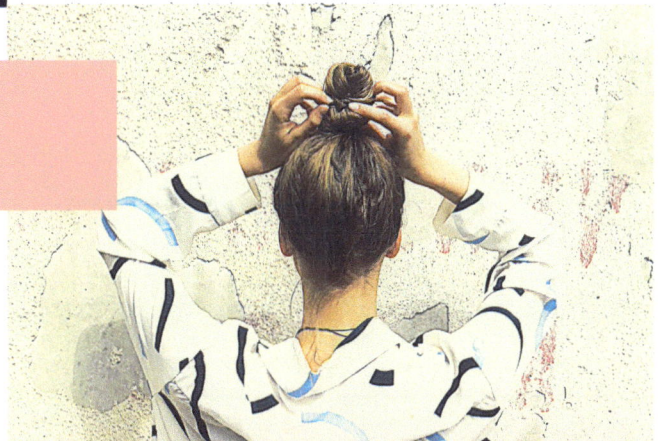

Deep and meaningful relationships play a vital role in overall well-being.

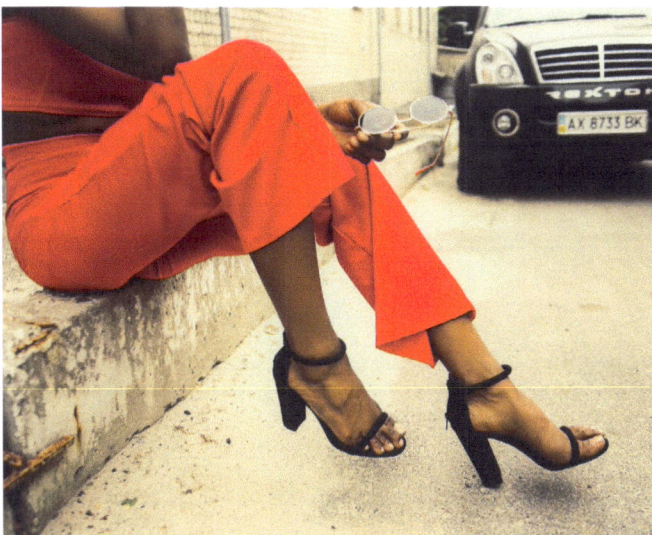

www.ingramcontent.com/pod-product-compliance
Lightning Source LLC
Chambersburg PA
CBHW060844270326
41933CB00003B/186